Rania Kaddoussi
Raoûa Naouar

Distinctive features of asthma in high school students

Rania Kaddoussi
Raoûa Naouar

Distinctive features of asthma in high school students

ScienciaScripts

Imprint

Cover image: www.ingimage.com

This book is a translation from the original published under ISBN 978-620-6-72605-0.

Publisher:
Sciencia Scripts
is a trademark of
Dodo Books Indian Ocean Ltd. and OmniScriptum S.R.L publishing group

120 High Road, East Finchley, London, N2 9ED, United Kingdom
Str. Armeneasca 28/1, office 1, Chisinau MD-2012, Republic of Moldova, Europe
Managing Directors: Ieva Konstantinova, Victoria Ursu
info@omniscriptum.com

Printed at: see last page
ISBN: 978-620-8-50301-7

CONTENTS

LIST OF ABBREVIATIONS

CHU: Centre Hospitalo-Universitaire

GINA: Global Initiative for Asthma

MMAS: Morisky Medication Adherence Scale

FEV1: forced expiratory volume second

CV: vital capacity Vital capacity

TCA: Allergic skin test

LABA: long-acting inhaled β2-adrenergics

WHO: World Health Organization

Chapter 1

INTRODUCTION

Asthma is a complex and common chronic inflammatory disease of the airways, characterized by bronchial hyperactivity [1].

In 2019, according to estimates by the World Health Organization (WHO), 262 million people will suffer from asthma, with a death toll of 461,000 [2]. Asthma is currently considered one of the most common chronic diseases in children [2,3].

In Tunisiaasthma affects 12% of children under the age of 15 [4], the main etiology being allergy. It is responsible for hospitalization rates 6.6% and emergency room use of 28.6% at least once a year [5]. This shows that asthma control was sub-optimal, and can be explained by the fact that adolescence is a sensitive and often problematic period of transition.

Being a high-school student and living with a chronic disease is hard enough: facing therapeutic constraints and physical limitations, it's also the time to be aware of the damage to your body and the inevitable confrontation with pathology [6]. This leads poor asthma control, high morbidity and mortality, and high asthma-related healthcare costs [6].

Thus, therapeutic education is essential in order to lead them to autonomy, hence the interest of our study with the following objectives

- Evaluating therapeutic compliance among high-school students with asthma and studying its determining factors

Chapter 2

PATIENTS AND METHODS

I. Features of the study

1. Type of study

This is a cross-sectional analytic study including adolescents followed at the Pneumology Department of the Fattouma Bourguiba University Hospital in Monastir during the period from 1996 to 2020.

2. Population of the study

❖ **Inclusion criteria:**

We included in our study patients meeting the following criteria:

- Age between 12 and 18
- Followed at the pneumology department of CHU Fattouma Bourguiba Monastir for at least 3 months.
- Confirmed asthma based on GINA diagnostic criteria [7].
- A confirmed allergic phenotype

❖ **Non-inclusion criteria:**

- Ages under 12 and over 18
- Mental disorders
- Asthma of non-allergic etiology

3. data collection

All patients recruited were asked to complete a pre-established questionnaire and a treatment adherence score (the Morisky score) (appendix 1).

This sheet includes :

- An interview to record patient demographics: identification, age, gender,
- Lifestyle habits and pathological antecedents: co-morbidities, family and personal atopy
- Asthma disease characteristics: age of onset, duration, seasonality, level of asthma control according to GINA criteria, number of hospitalizations/year.
- Asthma treatment: the therapeutic regimen
- Compliance was assessed using the Morisky questionnaire or the MMAS score.

All participants underwent spirometry to assess the severity of bronchial obstruction.

4. Definition of variables

4.1. The level of control of asthma

Assessment of the level of asthma control over the previous 4 weeks was based on the GINA asthma control criteria, which include frequency of daytime symptoms, nocturnal awakening, frequency of use of rescue medication and presence of physical activity limitations [7].

Three levels of control are defined:

- Well-controlled asthma: no criteria met
- Partially controlled asthma: 1 to 2 criteria present
- Uncontrolled asthma: 3 or more criteria present

4.2. Confirmation of allergy

The allergic phenotype asthma was retained if one or more of these criteria were present:

- Allergic skin test (TCA) positivity to one or more allergens, using the Prick test method.
  - The test is performed by rubbing a drop of each standardized allergen solution onto the anterior surface of both forearms, on skin already disinfected with alcohol.
  - Results are interpreted in relation to the positive control (histamine) and the negative control.
  - The test is said to be positive if the diameter of the papule obtained at the 15th minute is more than 3 millimeters greater than that of the negative control, or if the diameter of the papule is more than half that of the positive control.
- A serum specific immunoglobulin E assay is performed if there is a discrepancy between the clinically suspected allergen and results obtained from the APTT, or if the allergen is not available in APTT, or if APTT is uninterpretable or not feasible. A level above 0.35 IU for one or more allergens is considered significant. The technique used is RAST.

4.3. treatment stages

There are five levels of treatment: the steps are divided from 1 to 5, with two tracks depending on the rescue agent's choice (appendix 2) [7].

4.4. Level compliance

In this study, we used the 4-item Morisky score (MMAS-4) to assess asthma treatment adherence (Appendix 1). To each item, the patient responds with "oui " or "non " and the response will be scored 0 or 1.

II. Analysis statistics

Data entry and statistical analysis were carried out using the SPSS version 20.

Quantitative variables were expressed as means± their standard deviations

Qualitative variables were expressed as numbers and percentages.

To compare means between two independent samples, we used Student's T-test.

To compare percentages, Pearson's chi-square test was used independent series, and in the event of non-validity, Fisher's two-tailed test was used.

For the various statistical tests used, a significance threshold was set at 0.05.

Chapter 3

RESULTS

1. Characteristics of the population studied

1.1. Characteristics epidemiological

Four hundred and ninety-one patients were included in this study.
The mean age of the patients was 15.27 ± 1.88 years.
Males predominated (56.), with a sex ratio of 1.29 (Figure 1).

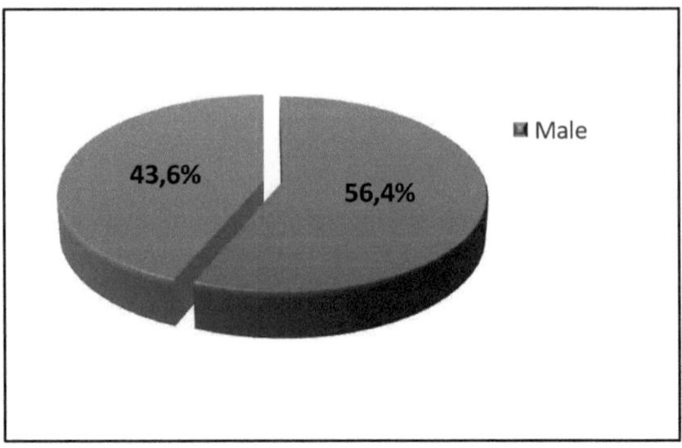

Figure 1: Distribution of study population by gender

1.2. Characteristics of asthmatic disease

The mean age of onset of asthma was 11.48± 4.08 years. The average duration of asthma was 39.95 ± 41.35 months.

Family atopy was found in 235 adolescents (48.1%).

Allergic manifestations other than asthma (rhinitis, conjunctivitis) were noted in 404 patients (82.3%).

Asthma was mild in 183 patients (37.3%), moderate in 300 (61.1%) and severe in 8 (1.6%).

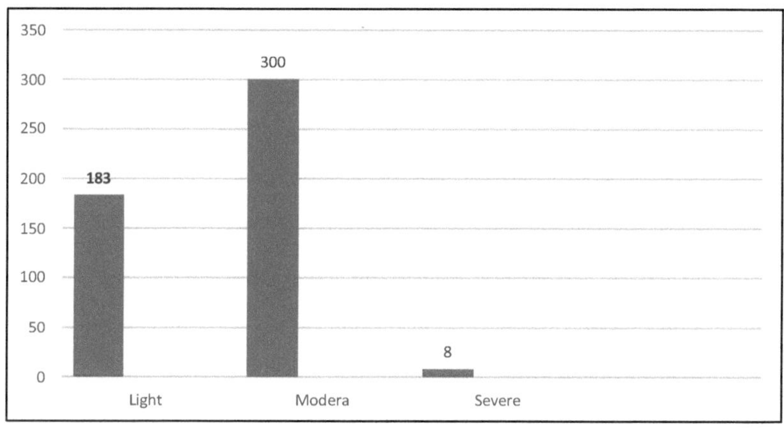

Figure 2: Initial asthma classification

Ventilatory exploration was performed by simple spirometry.

A reversibility test was performed in patients with obstructive ventilatory disorders. Mean FEV1 was 2920.65±810.79 ml (90.60±18.59%) with a mean FEV1/CV ratio of 91.11±59.81%.

The allergological workup showed that the pneumallergens involved were mainly house dust mites (338 cases).

1.3. Treatments

Asthma management in our series was based on medical and etiological treatment (desensitization, eviction,) (Table 1).

Table 1: Treatment allergic asthma adolescents

Treatment	N(%)
Inhaled corticoids	350(71,2)
LABA+CI	141(28,7%)
Antileukotriene	115(23,4)
Systemic corticosteroid therapy	4(0,8)
Specific immunotherapy	92(18,7)

1.4. Compliance

The majority of patients (318 or 64.8%) were considered compliant with asthma treatment according to the Morisky score (figure 3).

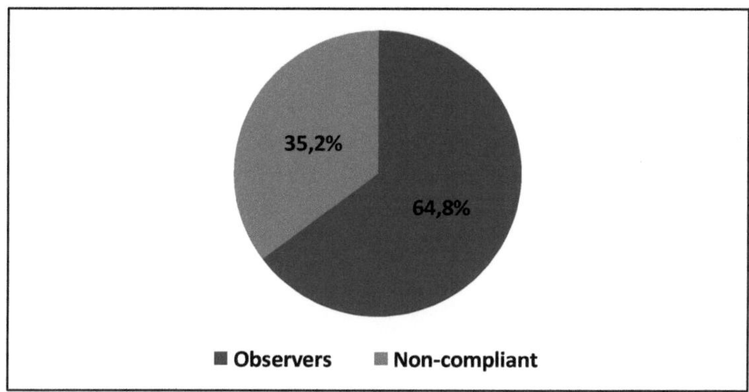

Figure 3: Distribution of patients according therapeutic compliance

1.5 Level of asthma control and evolution

The follow-up of our patients enabled us assess level of asthma control according to the GINA criteria for asthma control. Indeed, 357 patients (72.7%) were well controlled (figure 4).

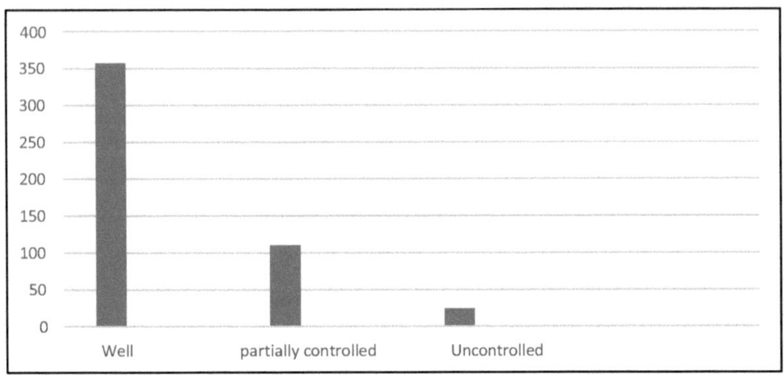

Figure 4: Level of asthma control

Among the high-school students hospitalized in the pulmonology department for acute asthma exacerbations, 16 patients were admitted only once, and only two adolescents had three hospitalizations.

Two patients required an intensive care unit stay for severe acute asthma.

2. Study analytical

2.1 Factors compliance therapy

We sought to identify factors associated with non-adherence to treatment in high-school students with asthma, based on a univariate study.

2.1.1 Patient factors

Female high school students and those with no personal history of atopy had poor compliance, with a significant difference as shown in Table 2.

Table 2: Patient-related factors therapeutic compliance

Factors	P
Age	NS
Gender	0,016
Personal history atopy	0,02

2.1.2 Factors linked to pathology

Factors linked to asthma pathology that were significantly correlated with the level of therapeutic adherence included: severity of asthma and obstructive syndrome, seasonality and number of allergens.

> =2 (Table 3).

Table 3: Pathology-related factors therapeutic compliance

Factors	**Compliance therapeutic**		**P**
	Yes (318)	**No (173)**	
Age of asthma onset (years)			
average± standard deviation	11.56± 4.14	11.33± 3.98	
Age of asthma (months)			
mean± standard deviation	41,08± 41,76	37.86± 40.61	
Severity (n,%)			
severe	2(25%)	6(75%)	0,01
FEV1 (mL)			
average± standard deviation	2770.47± 792.53	3011.29± 809.61	0,002
Seasonal asthma (n,%)			
perennial	232(67,4%)	112(32,6%)	
Summer and spring	38(48,1%)	41(51,9%)	0,01
Winter	48(70,6%)	20(29,4%)	
Number of allergens >=2			
(n,%)	216(89,3%)	26(10,7%)	0,046

Tissue eosinophilia (IU)

average± standard deviation 0.44± 0.49 0,±

0,42 0,01

Treatment stage<= 3 (n,%)		
Stage 2	38(36,5%) 66(63,5%)	
10-3		
Stage 3	69(52,7%) 62(47,3%)	

Chapter 4

DISCUSSION

Despite continuous progress in the health field and the multiplicity of therapeutic strategies, asthma still represents a real burden for several reasons, particularly among high-school students, whose mortality rate continues to rise [8,9]. Poor compliance with treatment is one of these reasons [1,8,10,11]. In this study, we propose therapeutic compliance among asthmatic adolescents, and to identify the determining factors of non-adherence and its consequences.

Our results showed a mean age of the participants of 15.27± 1.88 years [12 - 18 years] and a sex ratio of 1.29. The mean age of onset of asthma symptoms was 11.48 ± 4.08 years, with a mean course of 39.95 ± 41.35 months. One hundred and thirty-eight high-school students had mild asthma, and only 8 patients had severe asthma. Ventilatory testing revealed a mean FEV1 of 2920.65 ± 810.79 ml. A total of 318 or 64.8% of patients were considered compliant with asthma treatment.

Estimates of compliance rates vary from study to study. Rates of non-adherence to asthma treatment are generally between 30% and 70% [12]. Tunisian data on asthma in high-school students are very limited, if not non-existent.

Studies of childhood asthma using electronic compliance monitoring have shown average adherence rates well below 75%, with up to half of studies reporting rates of 50

% or even less [13,14].

This sub-optimal adherence may be significantly associated with worsening asthma, with the risk of unnecessary therapeutic escalation, increased school absenteeism and impaired quality of life in adolescents [15,16,17,18].

In our series, we noted a slight male predominance (56.4%) in our patients. A gender discrepancy in the prevalence of asthma has been reported in the literature. Infantile asthma affects boys more than girls, but the trend reverses after puberty [19].

In the International Study of Asthma and Allergies in Childhood (ISAAC), considered the most comprehensive international survey of asthma to date, which included 257,800 children aged 6-7 in 38 countries, and 463,801 children aged 13-14 in 56 countries, prevalence of asthma was higher in boys in the 6-7 age group, while girls had a higher prevalence in the 13-14 age group. There were considerable variations between countries [20]. Our study showed a male predominance (56.4%), which is not in line with these findings. This can be explained by the fact that our service is mainly dedicated to the population of the governorate of Monastir, where the number of male adolescents is higher than that of girls in the 14-19 age group during the period of our study (1995-2020) [21].

Affecting both boys and girls, asthma remains a disruptive factor in teenagers' quality of life, making research into the factors involved in asthma control an essential strategy for reducing the adverse health effects and financial burden of the disease [22].

Studies of asthma control have shown that most asthmatics are uncontrolled [23,24]. In particular, the American Real-World Evaluation of Asthma Control and Treatment (REACT) study of 1,812 patients with moderate to severe asthma concluded that asthma control was not achieved in 55% of patients [25,26]. The AIRMAG study [27], carried out for the first time in North Africa and which also included Tunisia, showed that 48% of asthmatics in our country were uncontrolled. These studies mainly included adults, but the results were similar to those seen in adolescent

asthmatics. In our sample, 27.3% of patients had uncontrolled asthma.
Pharmacological treatments for asthma, if used correctly, offer good symptom control and improved quality of life for patients. Therapeutic education ensures this control by educating asthma patients about their condition, how their medication works and how to use it correctly. It also helps patients acquire or maintain skills in asthma disease management. [28].

A meta-analysis published in 2017, including 270 randomized controlled trials, focused on therapeutic adherence and demonstrated that asthma self-management training optimizes asthma-related clinical outcomes, with a significant reduction in emergency room visits, unscheduled medical visits and admissions, and an improvement in asthma control and quality of life. [29].

Another controlled trial involving 126 patients presenting to emergency departments for acute asthma attacks, studied the effect of educational interventions limited to simply checking that inhalers were being taken and giving a self-action plan during the emergency department consultation, and the effect of structured, self-management-focused education delivered in several sessions. After 6 months, only self-management education led to a significant improvement medication use, patient quality of life, PEFs and a reduction in the number of unscheduled consultations [30].

In the literature, a number of methods assessing compliance with asthma therapy have been reported, but none of them meet acceptable criteria of feasibility and reliability [31]. These methods can be divided into direct and indirect methods [32].

Direct methods are expensive and often invasive. They are also difficult to apply on a large scale and ethically questionable, since they are often regarded by the patient as a means of supervision [32]. These methods include pill counting, monitoring via electronic pillboxes and measurement

of serum drug concentration levels. Nevertheless, bioassay appears to be the only direct method that accurately assesses medication compliance. However, this method of assessment becomes more difficult and complicated in the case of polymedications, given the complexity of therapeutic regimens and the differences in the timing of drug intake [32].
Indirect methods include several measures such as proportion of days covered (PDC), medication possession ratio (MPR), composite adherence score and the Morisky Medication Adherence Scale (MMAS), which is the most commonly used method. This multiplicity of measures, although simple and inexpensive, makes comparison between studies increasingly difficult [32]. According to many authors, self-reported methods have the potential to overestimate adherence.
In the case of asthma, no questionnaire has yet been validated in French or Arabic to assess compliance with background treatment. The Morisky questionnaire was used to assess compliance in our series.
Based on a univariate study, we investigated the factors associated with poor therapeutic adherence including medication compliance and follow-up compliance. Our results showed that the factors significantly associated with poor therapeutic adherence were female gender, mild obstructive syndrome and perennial symptomatology, which can be explained by false confidence felt by asthmatics with non-persistent mild symptomatology. Indeed, Dal Negro noted in a retrospective observational study of adolescent asthmatics referred to the pulmonary unit of the specialized medical center, in Italy, over a 12-month period, that compliance was poor in patients with mild to moderate asthma [33]. Most of the reasons given for non-adherence in the case of mild asthma were the lack of need felt by adolescents with asthma for daily treatment, overestimation of asthma control and lack of perception of the effect of the condition on daily activities. However, severe asthma attacks can occur in uncontrolled

intermittent asthma, contributing to the persistence of the disease.

Age of onset and duration of asthma were not related to therapeutic compliance. This is reminiscent of the results of a cohort study on European Community Respiratory Health (ECRHS), which included 971 asthmatic subjects from 12 countries who participated in both the ECRHS-I (1990- 94) and ECRHS-II (1998-2002) follow-up studies, and which concluded that age of onset and duration of asthma were not significant determinants of improved or persistent compliance with asthma treatment [34]. This may be explained by the fact that the earlier the onset of asthma and the longer it lasts, the less adherent the adolescent becomes to treatment, and the more frequent the forgetfulness.

This lack of compliance is a factor in poor asthma control and exacerbations, and may play a role in the majority of asthma deaths [35,36,37]. Milgrom et al. showed that median adherence to inhaled corticosteroid therapy, as measured by electronic monitoring, in poorly controlled children was 13%, compared with adherence in children without severe exacerbations [38]. In addition, avoidable factors have been identified in the majority of asthma-related deaths including adequate therapeutic education. In a study of the circumstances preceding 90 deaths asthma attacks, 77% of patients failed to identify the severity of their attack and delayed seeking medical help [36]. This study found that the risk of mortality decreased when the patient received good therapeutic education. [35,39].

This underlines the importance of proper therapeutic education for asthmatic adolescents. In France, there are several "Asthma Schools" dedicated to the therapeutic education (ETP) of asthmatic children.

B. Lesourd et al conducted a study at the "Alizée" Asthma School in Toulouse, and found that the number of emergency room visits in 6 months was twice as low (15% versus 30%) after the education sessions, and that no more children were admitted for their asthma, even though 23% of them had been hospitalized in the 6 months prior to the sessions [40].

Another French study demonstrated a rapid beneficial effect of ETP, after 3 to 4 sessions, on quality of life and level of asthma control [41].

Indeed, these results found that these programs were significantly associated with improved disease self-management and lung function, with fewer emergency room visits and less school absenteeism.

Chapter 5

Study limits

Our work has certain limitations, mainly of a methodological nature, which could be a source of bias.

The monocentric and cross-sectional nature of our study is one of its limitations. , this type study presents difficulties in interpreting associations, which makes it impossible to confirm the existence of a causal link between variables.

-Adherence assessment methods are also sources of bias. In fact, direct methods are very intrusive, unlike indirect methods, which make it difficult to obtain objective results. What's more, in our study, the questions were asked by the physician prescribing the treatment, which may amplify the self-reported overestimation due to patients' desire to "please".

Study highlights

In Tunisia, only a limited number of studies have been carried out therapeutic compliance asthmatic adolescents, and our study is one of them.

Furthermore, our study will enable us in the future to strengthen strategies for optimizing therapeutic education for asthmatic adolescents followed up in our department, in order to improve level of control their disease.

Therapeutic education for asthmatic adolescents

Organization:

- Shared time between teenagers and parents will be avoided.
- Based on an accelerated program, it will be divided into three 2.5-hour group sessions.
- Carried out by a multidisciplinary team trained therapeutic education in the form of a therapeutic education campaign for asthma in adolescents.
- The effects of tobacco and other inhalant irritants will be discussed with adolescents.

The first session :

At the beginning of the session

- An initial video-sharing session with the teenagers' parents
- A presentation between the team and the teenager
- An educational diagnosis
- Therapeutic education

- Presentation of the educational diagnostic tool :

The assessment of adolescents' knowledge and skills in relation to asthmatic disease will be carried out in the form of a paper-drawing game. Each small paper contains two questions.

Game terms and conditions:

The papers will be placed in a jar. The evaluation will be done individually, to avoid any comparison or judgment by the teenagers. The teenager will draw the papers at random and try to answer the questions. One point will be awarded for each correct answer. An initial evaluation will be carried out at the end of the first session, and each teenager will have his or her own sheet.

Open-ended questions are preferred, as they offer a personalized perception. Questions will cover :

- **Biomedical dimensions of pathology :**

-Age of onset, duration and severity of asthma.

-Other pathological antecedents.

-Reasons for hospitalization and frequency.

- **Socio-educational dimensions :**

-Leisure and activities of daily life

-Family and social environment.

- **Cognitive dimensions :**

-Beliefs about :

Mechanisms of asthma

Factors that trigger asthma attacks

treatments work and their effectiveness The

benefits of therapeutic education

- **Psycho-affective dimensions :**

-Assessing the stage in pathology acceptance process

-Reactions to an asthma attack

-What is the adolescent patient's project?

- Therapeutic education :

The content of therapeutic education will be divided into three areas, according to the French national agency for health accreditation and evaluation (ANAES) [28]:

- **Knowledge:** Understand your pathology, identify the factors leading to an acute attack, its signs of severity and how to prevent it, understand how to take your medication.

- **Skills:** Knowing the peak flow meter, inhalation techniques, controlling breathing in different situations.

- **Attitudes:** Being able to express one's experiences, to know the behaviors adapted to the different symptoms with or without the help of one's entourage, to know how to manage one's pathology according to one's activities and projects, to know the behaviors adapted to prevent asthma attacks.

Methodology and resources :

The education sessions will be divided according to age into two groups: one with the 7 youngest and one with the 7 oldest.

The sessions will be based on the following ANAES guidelines: respiratory physiology, asthmatic disease, asthma attacks and their treatment, disease-modifying therapy, peak flow.

At the start of each new session, provide a reminder of what has already been learned, and clearly present each objective to be achieved, which will be repeated at the end of the session.

Second session 2 weeks later: duration 2h30

Safety" objectives:

Using a drawing or text, explain the first signs of a crisis and the triggers.

Explain the need to carry a bronchodilator and what to do in the event of an acute attack.

Wear a scarf in cold weather.

Know the difference between crisis treatment and disease-modifying therapy. Know the effects of tobacco and other inhaled irritants on asthma control.

At the end, an evaluation will be made through an educational report.

Third session two months later: lasting 2.5 hours

Hold round-table discussions with parents to review the first two sessions and put them into practice.

For adolescents, complete with PEF measurement and interpretation. Finally, provide the patient with a report for the attending physician.

Chapter 6

CONCLUSION

Asthma is a common chronic disease affecting some 262 million people worldwide, and its prevalence is still rising. This makes it a real health burden, particularly among high-school students, whose morbidity-mortality rate remains fairly high. One of its causes is poor compliance with treatment, which is generally low among children and high-school students.

It's clear that different asthma management strategies exist and are updated every year, but their effectiveness in improving adherence is still lacking.

In light of our findings, new approaches to understanding and improving asthma medication adherence high school students are urgently needed. Future interventions should be modifiable according to individual preferences, and should aim to provide practical reminders for both the adolescent and his or her parents.

, parental involvement should be further explored in consultation by questioning parents about their beliefs regarding asthma therapies and exploring their knowledge of practical disease management. Similarly, making adolescents capable self-assessing asthma control and the severity of an acute attack, as well as mastering self-management of their disease, is one of the main objectives of TVE.

Finally, it should be pointed out that Tunisia's experience in evaluating therapeutic education and setting up educational programs aimed solely at teenagers is still deficient, which is why the creation of "asthma schools" is urgently needed.

REFERENCES

1. Boinet T, Leroy-David C. Asthma in adults. Actual Pharm. Feb 2021;60(603):13-7.

2. Asthma [Internet]. [cited 6 Jan 2023]. Available from: https://www.who.int/fr/news-room/fact-sheets/detail/asthma

3. Bourdin A, Doble A, Godard P. The Asthma Insights and Reality in the Maghreb (AIRMAG) study: perspectives and lessons. Respir Med. Dec 2009;103:S38-48.

4. Sonia T, Meriem M, Yacine O, Nozha BS, Nadia M, Bechir L, et al. Prevalence of asthma and rhinitis in a Tunisian population. Clin Respir J. Feb 2018;12(2):608-15.

5. El Ftouh M, Yassine N, Benkheder A, Bouacha H, Nafti S, Taright S, et al. Paediatric asthma in North Africa: the Asthma Insights and Reality in the Maghreb (AIRMAG) study. Respir Med. Dec 2009;103:S21-9.

6. Jacquin P, Levine M. Compliance difficulties in chronic diseases during adolescence: understanding for action. Arch Pediatrie. Jan 2008;15(1):89-94.

7. Global Initiative for Asthma.Global Strategy for Asthma Management and Prevention, 2021.[Online]. [Accessed 05/01/2022], Available URL: https://ginasthma.org/wp-content/uploads/2021/05/GINA-Main-Report-2021- V2-WMS.pdf

8. De Simoni A, Horne R, Fleming L, Bush A, Griffiths C. What do adolescents with asthma really think about adherence to inhalers? Insights from a qualitative analysis of a UK online forum. BMJ Open. June 2017;7(6):e015245.

9. Penza-Clyve SM, Mansell C, McQuaid EL. Why Don't Children Take Their Asthma Medications? A Qualitative Analysis of Children's Perspectives on Adherence. J Asthma. Jan 2004;41(2):189-97.

10. Mäkelä MJ, Backer V, Hedegaard M, Larsson K. Adherence to

inhaled therapies, health outcomes and costs in patients with asthma and COPD. Respir Med. Oct 2013;107(10):1481-90.

12. Rand CS, Wise RA. Measuring Adherence to Asthma Medication Regimens. Am J Respir Crit Care Med. Feb 1994;149(2_pt_2):S69-76.

13. Kaplan A, Price D. Treatment Adherence in Adolescents with Asthma. J Asthma Allergy. Jan 2020;Volume 13:39-49.

14. Morton RW, Everard ML, Elphick HE. Adherence in childhood asthma: the elephant in the room. Arch Dis Child. 1 Oct 2014;99(10):949-53.

15. Fitzgerald D. Non-compliance in adolescents with chronic lung disease: causative factors and practical approach. Paediatr Respir Rev. 1 Sep 2001;2(3):260-7.

16. Burg GT, Covar R, Oland AA, Guilbert TW. The Tempest: Difficult to Control Asthma in Adolescence. J Allergy Clin Immunol Pract. May 2018;6(3):738-48.

17. Meltzer LJ, Ullrich M, Szefler SJ. Sleep Duration, Sleep Hygiene, and Insomnia in Adolescents with Asthma. J Allergy Clin Immunol Pract. sept 2014;2(5):562-9.

18. Jonsson M, Bergström A, Egmar AC, Hedlin G, Lind T, Kull I. Asthma during adolescence impairs health-related quality of . J Allergy Clin Immunol Pract. janv 2016;4(1):144-146.e2.

19. Arathimos R, Granell R, Henderson J, Relton CL, Tilling K. Sex discordance in asthma and wheeze prevalence in two longitudinal cohorts. Lee YL, editor. PLOS ONE. 25 Apr 2017;12(4):e0176293.

21. en.zhujiworld.com. World statistics 2023 [Internet]. [cited March 2, 2023]. Available from: https://fr.zhujiworld.com/

22. Nunes C, Pereira AM, Morais-Almeida M. Asthma costs and social impact. Asthma Res Pract. Dec 2017;3(1):1.

23. Mintz M, Gilsenan AW, Bui CL, Ziemiecki R, Stanford RH,

Lincourt W, et al. Assessment of asthma control in primary care. Curr Med Res Opin. 1 Oct 2009;25(10):2523-31.

24. Demoly P, Paggiaro P, Plaza V, Bolge SC, Kannan H, Sohier B, et al. Prevalence of asthma control among adults in France, Germany, Italy, Spain and the UK. Eur Respir Rev. June 1, 2009;18(112):105-12.

25. Peters SP, Jones CA, Haselkorn T, Mink DR, Valacer DJ, Weiss ST. Real- world Evaluation of Asthma Control and Treatment (REACT): Findings from a national Web-based survey. J Allergy Clin Immunol. June 2007;119(6):1454-61.

26. Barcala FJG, Nuevo J, Caamaño-Isorna F. Factors Associated with Asthma Control in Primary Care Patients in Spain: The CHAS study. Arch Bronconeumol.

27. Benkheder A, Bouacha H, Nafti S, Taright S, El Ftouh M, Yassine N, et al. Control of asthma in the Maghreb: results of the AIRMAG study. Respir Med. Dec 2009;103:S12-20.

28. HAS (2013-01-25). Adult asthma education- Recommendationsavailable on :https://www.hassante.fr/upload/docs/application/pdf/education_adulte_asthma ti que_recommendations.pdf

29. for the PRISMS and RECURSIVE groups, Pinnock H, Parke HL, Panagioti M, Daines L, Pearce G, et al. Systematic meta-review of supported self-management for asthma: a healthcare perspective. BMC Med. Dec 2017;15(1):64.

30. Côté J, Bowie DM, Robichaud P, Parent JG, Battisti L, Boulet LP. Evaluation of Two Different Educational Interventions for Adult Patients Consulting with an Acute Asthma Exacerbation. Am J Respir Crit Care Med. May 1, 2001;163(6):1415-9.

31. de Blicj J. Therapeutic compliance in asthmatic children. Rev Mal Respir. Apr 2007;24(4):419-25.

32. Pednekar PP, Ágh T, Malmenäs M, Raval AD, Bennett BM, Borah BJ, et al. Methods for Measuring Multiple Medication Adherence: A Systematic Review-Report of the ISPOR Medication Adherence and Persistence Special Interest Group. Value Health. Feb 2019;22(2):139-56.

33. Dal Negro RW, Turco P. Effects of Adherence to Once-Daily Treatment on Lung Function, Bronchial Hyperreactivity and Health Outcomes in Adolescents with Mild-to-Moderate Asthmoka: A Twelve-Month Survey. Children. Dec 2022;9(12):1854.

34. Corsico AG, Cazzoletti L, de Marco R, Janson C, Jarvis D, Zoia MC, et al. Factors affecting adherence to asthma treatment in an international cohort of young and middle-aged adults. Respir Med. June 2007;101(6):1363-7.

35. Ducharme FM, Parent AM, Verreault N, Michaud L, Fontaine R, Flibotte J, et al. ADHERENCE TO TREATMENT IN ASTHMATIC TEENAGERS: PISTES DE SOLUTION POUR LE RÉSEAU DE SANTÉ QUÉBÉCOIS. 2009;

36. D'Amato G, Vitale C, Molino A, Stanziola A, Sanduzzi A, Vatrella A, et al. Asthma-related deaths. Multidiscip Respir Med. Dec 2016;11(1):37.

37. Harrison B, Stephenson P, Mohan G, Nasser S. An ongoing Confidential Enquiry into asthma deaths in the Eastern Region of the UK, 2001-2003. Prim Care Respir J. Dec 2005;14(6):303-13.

38. Milgrom H, Bender B, Ackerson L, Bowrya P, Smith B, Rand C. Noncompliance and treatment failure in children with asthma☆☆☆★ . J Allergy Clin Immunol. Dec 1996;98(6):1051-7.

39. Barton CA, McKenzie DP, Walters EH, Abramson MJ, The Victorian Asthma Mortality Stud. Interactions Between Psychosocial Problems and Management of Asthma: Who Is at Risk of Dying? J Asthma. Jan 2005;42(4):249-56.

40. Lesourd B, Juchet A, Broué-Chabbert A, Colineaux H. À l'École de l'Asthme... Bilan et évaluation d'une éducation thérapeutique. Rev Fr Allergol. oct 2014;54(6):438-50.

41. Beydon N, Robbe M, Lebras MN, Marchand V, Périès MA, Alberti C, et al. Quality of life, asthma control, cotininuria and therapeutic education in asthmatic children. Santé Publique. 2012;24(2):105-19.

APPENDICES

Appendix 1: MMAS score

Morisky Medication Adherence Scale (MMAS)

MMAS	Oui	Non
Vous arrive-t-il d'oublier de prendre votre traitement ?		
Vous arrive-t-il de ne pas faire attention aux jours auxquels vous prenez votre traitement ?		
Si vous vous sentez parfois moins bien lorsque vous prenez votre traitement, cessez-vous de le prendre ?		
Lorsque vous vous sentez mieux, arrêtez-vous parfois de prendre votre traitement ?		

Points attribués à chaque item
Oui = 1 Non = 0

Patient très observant = 0
Patient modérément observant = 1 ou 2
Patient non observant = 3 ou 4

Appendix 2: Stages in the treatment allergic asthma adolescents

Step	Processing track 1	Processing track 2
1	β2LDA on demand	-
2	Low-dose IC alone	
3	Medium-dose CI- β2LDA	Dose CI medium-anti leukotriene
4	High dose CI- β2LDA	Dose CI average-β2LDA-anti leukotriene
5	High-dose CI -β2LDA-anti leukotriene	CI à dose maximum-β2LDA-anti leukotriene

Summary

Introduction: Asthma in high school students is often under-diagnosed, which can affect their academic performance. High school students with asthma may face challenges related to the management of their condition, especially in the school environment. We conducted this study investigate the particularities asthma in high school students.

Patients and methods: analytical cross-sectional study conducted at the Pneumology Department of the Fattouma Bourguiba University Hospital in Monastir .

Results :

The mean age of onset of asthma was 11.48± 4.08 years. The average duration of asthma was 39.95 ± 41.35 months.

Allergic manifestations in addition to asthma (rhinitis, conjunctivitis) were noted in 404 patients (82.3%). Asthma was mild in 183 patients (37.3%), Asthma was moderate in 300 patients (61.1%) and severe in 8 (1.6%). 357 patients (72.7%) were well controlled.

Conclusion: Asthma is a common condition in high school students, which can lead to absences and reduced performance. School pressure and sports activities can exacerbate symptoms, making disease management crucial.

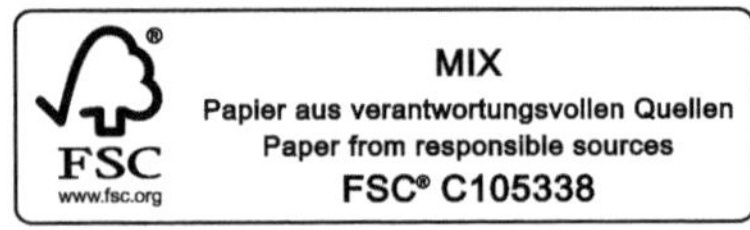

Printed by Books on Demand GmbH, Norderstedt / Germany